Declutter Your Mind

Learn How To Free Yourself From Mental Clutter And Live A Richer Life Today!

Book Description

This world we live in is so full of distractions, it's amazing we can keep anything straight. When it falls to you to take care of the deadlines at work or in college, tend to the bills and payments that are constantly coming up, and keep up with the daily family obligations you have, your mind can easily become overwhelmed.

Combine those physical duties with stress, overthinking, and continually trying to maintain your sanity – and you have a recipe for disaster.

It's no secret that most of the adults in today's world feel overburdened and worn out, and it's even more well-known that many adults in today's world are taking some form of medication to help them cope with the mental stress they are placed under on a daily basis.

Forgetfulness, headaches, and feeling like you will never be able to keep up – let alone relax – are common feelings in the modern adult. But, they don't have to be.

With the right mindset, you can free your mind of all the excess stress and worry that you are currently experiencing – and that's where this book comes in.

In it, you are going to earn the secret to decluttering your mind, and you will be able to free yourself of all those extra things that are weighing you down. As a result, you'll find the stress melt away, the anxiety fade, and you will be able to face life with a renewed freshness you've only dreamed of.

This book holds the secret to giving you the ultimate peace, and by utilizing these proven methods, you will give yourself both mental freedom and peace of mind.

- **Learn how to declutter the junk from your mind and live fully**

- **Use proven step-by-step methods to clear your mind and focus**

- **Experience a host of health benefits as you lower negativity and stress**

- **And much, much more!**

Contents

Introduction

Drop the kids off at school. Mail the bills. Go to work. Hurry up with that project so you can catch up on the other. Do errands. It's time to go pick up the kids again. Did I mention you're going to need to run to the store to grab a few things so you can make dinner?

And if this wasn't bad enough, the entire day your mind is on other things:

"What is my boss going to think about the data entry?"

"Is my friend mad at me for that comment I made the other night? I didn't mean anything by it."

"What if I don't get that second check in time to make the house payment?"

And the list goes on.

If this sounds like you don't worry, you are not alone. Millions of men and women across the planet stress about life every single day, and a large percentage of those people wind up feeling overwhelmed, depressed, or with some form of illness that is induced by the stress they are dealing with.

Our bodies are directly connected to our minds, and the things we feel and stress about puts actual, physical stress on the bodies we live in. While a little stress is a good thing, too much of it results in the body breaking down.

You can't sleep well. You don't eat right. You lose the mental energy to handle the problems that arise in your day well. You get stuck in a vicious cycle of trying to stay on top, but the harder you try, the more you sink.

Sadly, without making a deliberate change in your mindset, this problem is only going to get worse. This could potentially lead to a variety of health problems down the road including stroke, heart problems, and even cancer.

But, there is hope.

Your mind is a powerful thing, and with determination, some simple steps, and a lot of practice, you can change the way you deal with the stress in your life. Get rid of all that excess clutter, and free yourself from the mental agony you must deal with on a daily basis.

With the proven methods outlined in this book, you're going to finally understand what it means to be mentally free, and you'll begin living life to the fullest. It's not expensive, it's not hard, and the changes are real.

Are you ready to break out of this vicious cycle you have been trapped in? Are you ready to take control of your life and live fully? Are you ready to make that change?

Excellent. Let's get started.

Chapter 1 – What is Mental Clutter?

Most people have heard the term mental clutter, but not everyone fully understands what that truly means. Some are very specific in what they consider to be mental clutter – worry, fear, thinking too much about a particular thing, etc. while others take on a broader view of what it is.

To put it simply, mental clutter is anything in your mind that is holding you back from being the person you wish to be, or living the life you want to live. It might be one or two large things that eat away at you day after day, or it might be comprised of many different little things that constantly remain in the back of your mind.

You may be able to pinpoint your own mental clutter at this very moment. As you read this you think to yourself, "Yes! I know exactly what my clutter is; I just need to know how to get rid of it!"

Or, you may be someone who has been struggling with all the adverse side effects of having mental clutter, and you are now hoping to both identify what your clutter is, and learn how to get rid of it.

The first step to solving any problem is knowing that you have it, and understanding what that problem is.

Whether you are a person who considers mental clutter to be a broad and sweeping category, or whether you consider each little aspect of the clutter in and of itself, it's a good idea to know what to watch for in your own mind. Identify each part of the problem, then deal with each part as it arises.

Worry – Worry is one of the most common forms of mental clutter. It's tied closely to fear and guilt. While worry is always future oriented, it can spring from guilt over things you have done in the past, or things you are currently struggling with in your life.

Many people mistakenly assume if they worry about something they then have the power to change what is going to happen. Deep down inside, we all know that this isn't true, yet it doesn't change the fact that worry is one of the number one things that keep people up at night.

This is not to say that you need to live a passive life. You will always be responsible for the decisions you make, and each day requires that you make a lot of different decisions. However, being prepared to make decisions and worrying about what is going to happen next are two incredibly different things.

Negativity – in all its various forms, negativity is one of the biggest things to steal your happiness and clutter your mind. Some people spend their days being negative about themselves – they don't like their body, their house, their partner, their job – but they also tell themselves that they don't deserve anything better, or they aren't worth more.

Others spend their days being negative about the rest of the world – they can't believe how people are driving, what people are wearing, that they were cut off at the grocery store, the people at their job – and the list goes on.

Then there are those who spend their time negatively thinking about and discussing the "big picture" – that is to say, the things that they don't have any control over but are greatly affected by. Politics, the weather, the economy, and anything else like these things fall into this category.

Once you have been infected with negativity, it isn't long before it consumes every aspect of your life. It is as though your brain is unable to talk about any topic without adding on some form of negativity along with it.

"It is a nice day, but I'm starting to get a sunburn."

"I do like the new law, but now a lot of people will probably break it."

"I have lost some weight, but I've still got so much to lose, I'll probably never get there."

"That was nice of that man to let me go first, but he probably thinks that I'm a jerk for taking him up on the offer."

Negativity is like a weed. Once it takes root, it holds on tight and spreads as quickly as possible.

Outward focus – Another form of mental clutter which plagues many in the world today is the clutter that is focused on outward things. This clutter is worried about what other people think, what other people want, and whether the individual is liked or considered popular.

This clutter is largely fed through social media and comparing oneself to other people. When this clutter takes root, it isn't going to matter what happens to you as a person, there are always going to be people who are better off, more attractive, more impressive, more successful, and the list goes on.

These are just a few of the broader categories of mental clutter, and each one is an umbrella for all kinds of other things you may experience or be struggling with. But, there is good news.

Regardless of the mental clutter you are currently facing, you have the ability to conquer it and change the way you think. Don't be fooled into thinking that any of these things are not a big deal. As I have said before, our bodies are directly tied to the state our mind is in, and if you don't take care of these things now, you may end up facing even more harmful side effects in the future.

Chapter 2 – Scientific Truth: The Side Effects of a Cluttered Mind (and the Benefits of a Clear One)

If you struggle with mental clutter, you are already aware of the physical side effects this has on your life. However, you may be surprised to learn just how far reaching these side effects can be. In this chapter, I am going to show you how many things you may experience when you struggle with mental clutter – and some of the things you will experience as soon as you get rid of it.

Insomnia and fatigue – You know the feeling. You lie awake for hours, either unable to fall asleep in the first place, or stay asleep once you have managed to fall asleep. You try various tips and tricks, but nothing seems to work. For hours every night, it's just you and the darkness pressing in on you.

You may drift off closer to morning, but inevitably that alarm goes off and you are forced to get up and push into your day – but you are far from rested as you do so.

Aches and pains, especially in your back and neck – It really doesn't seem to take much before your back and neck start to ache. This happens whether you lift heavy things or spend your day sitting in front of your desk.

Tylenol and Ibuprofen really don't seem to do much for these aches and pains, either.

Loss of appetite and stomach pain – Mealtimes roll around, and all you can think of is what you need to be doing, or worrying about something that is going to happen in the future. You don't eat much, and when you do, it's something that you hope is going to make you feel better (macaroni and cheese, pizza... the things we consider to be "comfort" foods.)

Weight gain or weight loss – Regardless of your daily routine you see weight either coming or going, and both times it's not in the healthy regard. You can either end up drastically overweight though you try your hardest to stick with a low calorie diet.

Or, you may find that you are losing weight in spite of your efforts to maintain. It's not healthy weight loss that leaves you feeling good about yourself, it's the sickly kind of weight loss that makes you even more unhappy than you were before.

Blotchy skin or acne – That perfect skin seems to be completely out of reach as you try your hardest to fight dark circles, acne, and uneven skin tones. It seems that you are using far more concealer than you used to, while at the back of your mind you worry that it's only going to get worse from here.

Constipation – You know you aren't eating right or eating well when you do, so you wonder how you are constipated all the time. Stress releases hormones into your body which causes all of your systems to go haywire, so if you are struggling with any kind of mental clutter, you can be certain that your bowel movements are going to shift in a way that you don't care for.

Extreme medical conditions – None of the symptoms we have looked at this far are fun to deal with, and many of them only worsen the anxiety you are already feeling. However, if you don't get this under control, worse things such as heart attack, stroke, or even cancers can develop.

There is an alarming amount of cancer that has been attributed to mental stress and anxiety – meaning cleaning your mind may reduce your chances of getting these debilitating illnesses drastically.

As I have said before, there is hope. Once you get mental clutter under control and rid yourself of the clutter that is currently overwhelming your mind, you

will notice an incredible change from all these symptoms.

Restful sleep – It's true. When you have a happy and uncluttered mind, not only are you going to fall asleep easier and stay asleep, but you're also going to reach the restful sleep stage, and wake up feeling ready to face the new day with enthusiasm.

Energy – That sluggishness you feel during the day is going to disappear, as will the feeling that it is only a matter of time before something goes wrong. You will feel capable of handling anything that arises, and face each problem with the attitude that you'll get it taken care of.

Healthy appetite – Decluttering your mind will declutter your life in other ways, too. Clean up your diet, and soon you aren't going to have cravings for that junk food that leaves you feeling miserable. Healthy eating and a healthy mind go hand in hand, and combined you will experience something else you have always wanted – a healthy weight.

Healthy weight loss or gain – When you have a clear, healthy mind, your body can't help but respond. Your skin will take on a healthy glow, and your weight will even out into a healthy area. Sure, you might still want to gain or lose to be where you want to be, but you're going to lose that sick look – and feeling – almost immediately.

A regular routine in your lifestyle – Healthy eating combined with a healthy mind is going to change the way your body functions. You will no longer be constipated, you will adjust to normal sleep cycles, and you will see other routine changes in the way your body performs.

For many, a new desire to work out and take care of themselves emerges, as well as a more regular eating pattern. It's remarkable how clean your lifestyle becomes when you clean up your mind.

Lowered risk of extreme medical illness – Just as stress and mental clutter increases the risk for heart attack, stroke, and cancer, decluttering your mind and living a mindful lifestyle reduces the risk for all these illnesses drastically.

Within days of beginning your new lifestyle, you are going to notice remarkable change in how you think and feel about life, and the random issues that arise in your day to day living.

As you can see from both these lists, the mind and the body are closely connected to each other.

Stress is a powerful component which will happily take over your life if you let it. As you know, there is a healthy level of stress to live with, but too much stress only leads to health problems.

In the chapters to come, I am going to show you easy and effective ways to get rid of this mental clutter, as well as how to keep it from coming back. It's going to take deliberate effort on your part. But trust me, it's all going to be worth it.

Chapter 3 – Eliminating the Source: Where Does Mental Clutter Come From?

One of the problems with mental clutter is the fact that it can come from anywhere. Many people struggle with different forms of mental clutter because everyone is different and thinks about life in different ways. However, one common thread that ties everyone with mental clutter together is the fact that once it is gone, it could easily come back if you allow it to.

Mental clutter is a thought pattern. It's not something that slips in one day and can be pushed out the next. In order to get rid of the mental clutter in your life, you must first identify the source of that clutter, then deal with the problem where it begins.

Although mental clutter can come from anywhere, there is only one way it can stay in your mind – and that's if you allow it to.

There are those who blame the world for their clutter. They would have their lives together if only their partner was better, or their parents weren't so nagging, or if they hadn't experienced something traumatic in their childhood. These people become so convinced that the clutter in their mind is being forced on them, they shrivel up and refuse to try anything to get rid of it.

This thought process is not unlike other forms of mental clutter, however, as many people believe themselves to be a victim of their circumstances.

People who have mental clutter often come home to a house that is filled with things they don't need. The house may or may not be clean, but it certainly isn't organized, and it certainly is filled with a variety of things that are taking up space – physical space in the house that translates to mental space in the mind.

Think about it. If you were to look around your house and honestly ask yourself how much of the stuff you had was there because you loved it and wanted it, or how much of the stuff you had was there because you feel like you can't live without it, you will be surprised.

Close your eyes for a second and imagine the houses you see on TV. Houses that you consider to be very nice houses, or houses that are owned by the wealthy. If there is one thing you should notice about these houses it isn't that the appliances are updated or that they have hardwood floors.

Even the size of the house is irrelevant. The one thing you should notice in all these homes is that there is a lot of bare space. Now, this is not to say that this is empty space – empty space implies that there should be something there when there is not. No, think of this as bare space. Space that is there because space is valuable.

To someone who is trying to get rid of mental clutter, it is important to understand the value of space.

Relationships and our living spaces aren't the only places where mental clutter can creep in, either.

In our modern lives, we as people tend to live in two worlds – the physical one and the digital one. Sure, we wake up and live our lives out in the physical world, but we spend most of our emotional and mental time in the digital world. Between social media, news stories, online communities and groups, and doing everything you can to paint yourself as having the perfect life, you are spending more of your time in a digital universe while your real life passes you by.

This is why you spend so much of your day feeling as though you are spinning your tires without ever going anywhere. You wake up, walk out of your cluttered room into your cluttered kitchen, fumble around trying to find the things you need for breakfast, while you mind is already on what is going on down at the office.

You check your social media and are bombarded with the drama and perfect life of others, then as the kids get up and join you at the breakfast table you are given a list of things you need to do to care for them and keep them happy.

Don't misunderstand, I am not implying that by having duties or a busy life that you are supposed to be unhappy. What I am saying is that few people understand how to manage the business in their lives, and thus end up living in unhappy situations that leave them feeling incredibly overwhelmed.

There are millions of people on the planet who have discovered the secret to decluttering their mental lives, and they are still living lives that demand a lot of work from them. The difference isn't that these people clocked out of what they were supposed to be caring for, the difference is that these people have discovered the secret of handling the things that arise on a daily basis without letting it creep into their mental well-being.

Clutter comes from everywhere, and it can strike at any time. There are some days it may be worse than others, but if you know how to handle clutter when it comes knocking on your mental door, you can rest assured you will never have to deal with it taking root in your mind and affecting your well-being ever again.

In the chapters to come, I am going to show you how to effectively handle each of the sources of clutter one by one, freeing your life both mentally and physically.

Chapter 4 – Setting Yourself Up for Success: The Uncluttered Home

At first, the concept of decluttering your home is a daunting challenge. If you think about each and every room you're going to need to go through, and the things you're going to need to go through in each of the rooms, you may feel that familiar mental clutter of anxiety creep into your mind.

But before you get overwhelmed by the thought of going through all these things, I want to encourage you to think about how nice your house is going to look when you are done. Think of the time you are going to save when you get ready for work in the morning, or when you get ready for bed at night.

You aren't going to have to hunt for your medications or makeup, because you'll know right where it is. You won't have to rifle through piles of clothing to find the outfit you wish to wear the next day – your closet will be clear and organized, ready for you to grab what you want and go.

Imagine what it would be like to never have to search for the TV remote or the game console controller. Or how nice it would be to walk in and out of your home without tripping over shoes or coats in the entryway. Yes, you might be feeling overwhelmed with all the things you need to do now, but in the end you're going to feel better and freer in your life.

Bathroom – As you begin your decluttering process, start in the bathroom. Go through all the cabinets and get rid of old medication, and place the medication you take on a regular basis in the front. Store the other medication you keep on hand in the back where you can easily find it, but where it is out of the way.

Go through your makeup and get rid of the old or anything you don't wear often. Organize based on how often you wear it, and keep it in its place. Get rid of all the excess things you don't use – shampoo, lotion, creams, etc. You like what you like, and if you don't like it, get rid of it.

Bedroom – Bedrooms tend to be the rooms in the house in which things that don't really have a place tend to end up. They are on shelves, under beds, in closets – taking up space when there is no reason to hold onto it in the first place.

Go through all bedrooms in your home, and get rid of anything that you don't truly love. Anything. It doesn't matter if there is sentimental value, who gave it to you, or where you got it. If you don't look at it and immediately love it, get rid of it.

Kitchen – After you have completely gone through the bedrooms, it is time to turn your attention to the kitchen. Go through the kitchen with the same ferocity you went through the bedrooms, and ruthlessly get rid of anything that you don't love.

Do you hate your dishes? Get rid of them and get ones that you do like. How many people are in your home? Do you really need three of the same kind of pan or pot? Get rid of the food that has been hiding in the back of the pantry for ages.

Get rid of the décor that your mother in law gave you but you never truly enjoyed. If you look at something and you don't love it, get rid of it.

Living room – Living rooms can be difficult to declutter as they tend to be a mix of use and décor. You want your living area to look nice, especially when you have company over, but you don't want to spend your time rifling through things to find what you are really looking for.

Go through your living room with the same "love it or lose it" mindset, and get rid of anything you see that you don't love. Even things such as your entertainment center or the shelves on the wall need to go if you are keeping them for any reason besides loving them.

Entryway – The idea of an organized entryway is something that a lot of people really want. To be able to find what they are looking for without having to waste a lot of time would be heaven for most people, and you, too, could have this if you take the time to clean up.

Pack away the items that are out of season, and make a "no shoe" or "one pair" only rule for shoes left by the front door. Designate and area for mail to go in and out, and find a place to store your keys. It's remarkable how little you really need in the entryway of your home, and how big of an effect the entryway has on you feeling organized or stressed.

Storage closets/garage – Storage closets and the garage are two more areas in which things tend to land and never be seen again. These are not places that are meant to hold onto the junk you just can't see yourself getting rid of, they are supposed to be used for the things that you love and enjoy but don't want in the main part of your house.

Go through your garage and storage closets with brutal honesty, and determine why you really are hanging onto those tennis rackets when you haven't played since high school.

There are some very specific things you can ask yourself as you go through your home. Be honest with your answers, and never hang onto anything because you feel like you should, or because a certain person gave it to you.

As you go through each room, and each item in each room, ask yourself the following questions:

- **Do I love this?**

- **Does this item bring me joy?**

- **Why am I keeping this item?**

- **Is this item useful?**

- **Is this item excessive (for example, you don't need 2 sets of measuring spoons in your kitchen)?**

- **Am I keeping this item for anyone else besides me?**

- **When was the last time I used this item?**

- **Would I miss this item if it wasn't here?**

It can be difficult ridding yourself of the extra things in your life, especially if you are keeping things out of obligation. But, once you give yourself permission to be free of the expectations of other people (and even yourself) you'll finally be able to go through your rooms and rid yourself of the excess things that are weighing you down.

Lose the need to fill each space you have in your home, and begin finding the value of bare space. Simply because there is a shelf in the room doesn't mean it needs to be filled. In fact, the wall may look better without the shelf or the things that were on it.

Fill your home with the things you love, and only the things you love. The rest is just extra that is taking up physical and mental space that you could much better use in other ways – even if it's just to enjoy the bare space.

Chapter 5 – Clutter Cluster: Decluttering Your Relationships

It's an odd thing that in our world full of social media and instant communication, people are having a harder time than ever maintaining relationships with other people. This includes both the people that are merely friends as well as your family and even your partner.

Regardless of the relationship, the clutter manifests itself in much the same way. Unresolved issues, grievances, annoyances, and the like tend to creep in, and are only dealt with during an argument or disagreement of some kind. What happens is that with over time these things reach the point that they begin to suffocate the relationship, making it incredibly difficult for both people to truly thrive and appreciate each other.

Women especially tend to have clutter in their relationships as they hold onto each little thing that hurts their feelings, but instead of bringing it up and saying so to the other person in the relationship, they store it away until they are upset about something else.

In this chapter, we are going to discuss how you can effectively declutter all your relationships, and live life at peace with those around you – without keeping track of the wrongs that have been done or how you feel about those wrongs.

Regardless of the kind of relationship you are trying to declutter, you are going to focus on the same methods. Depending on how close you are with the individual you wish to declutter a relationship with, or the nature of the decluttering, you're going to have to decide how much work is going to go into it.

The first step to decluttering any relationship is communication.

In a world of instant communication to anyone in the world, it's a wonder how bad we are at communicating with each other. Yet, if you want to declutter your life, communication is key.

Instead of bottling things up, express how you feel to the other person. Don't do this in an accusatory or defensive way, merely say how you feel. It's remarkable how far you can go with someone when you are willing to say what you are thinking, rather than bottling it up and only bringing it up later on when anger is involved.

After you learn to communicate well (and often) you are ready to move into the next step of relationship decluttering: setting boundaries.

It doesn't matter what kind of relationship you have with someone, there are always going to be boundaries. With your friends, you may need to establish times when they are able to call or drop by, and times when that is not ok. If your friend who is going through a divorce suddenly calls you and you are only a few minutes away from an important appointment, tell them so.

"I'm sorry I can't talk very long right now, but I will give you a call back in a couple hours and we can chat longer."

If you are struggling with boundaries with your parents, respectfully remind them that you are an adult, and you need to make your own way in life. Remind them that you love them and are happy they care about you, but stay firm.

"I understand your concern about me moving to another state, and I am so glad you love me enough to tell me that you are concerned, but I am an adult now, and I need to make some of my own decisions."

Perhaps the boundaries need to come into place with your partner. In a loving and trusting relationship, both individuals need to understand and respect the boundaries their partner has put in place.

"I love you more than anything, and I am always happy to see you, but I really could use a couple hours to myself right now to unwind from the day. Can I pick you up later this evening?"

Many people are so afraid of offending someone that they don't ever place any boundaries in their relationships, and they end up feeling suffocated and overwhelmed. Learn how to put boundaries in place, then stand by those boundaries without feeling guilty about meeting your own needs.

Be kind to everyone – It doesn't matter if you have been lifelong friends or if you have just met someone walking down the street. One of the greatest ways you can declutter (and remain decluttered) is to be kind to everyone. Don't get sucked into needless drama, and even more importantly – don't start drama with anyone.

There is enough drama taking place in this world. You don't have to start it or fuel it.

Don't get wrapped up in expectations – Many times issues come up in relationships isn't because of what the other person is or isn't doing, it is because of our expectations of what we think they should or shouldn't do. The only person on this planet whose actions you have any control over is your own, so stop placing your expectations on other people.

When you have decided someone else should behave a certain way, you are only setting them up for failure and yourself up for disappointment. Let go of your expectations and learn to love the people in your life for who they are, not for who you think they should be.

Let go of the toxic people in your life – There are some instances when you simply can't win, and it's time to walk away. Analyze the relationships you are currently facing in your life, and be honest about the toxic people. It's better to simply walk away from these relationships than it is to try to stick with them, because some relationships just aren't going to give you the fulfillment they should.

You will learn as you declutter your relationships that much of the happiness in the relationship doesn't have much to do with the other person or people involved.

Instead of focusing on how they are there to make you happy, focus on what you can do in any given relationship to be easy to get along with. This is not to say that you need to do anything others want to keep them happy, but it does erase the mental record and expectations you tend to build over time.

Relationship decluttering can be one of the most difficult aspects of your life to declutter (and keep decluttered) but as with the other parts of your life, with practice you'll get the hang of things. It's been said that you teach other people how they ought to treat you, so learn to teach others to respect you while you do your best to be a good friend to them.

Chapter 6 – Cleanliness From the Inside Out: Decluttering Your Digital World

Although there are many wonderful things that have come from modern technology, it didn't come without a cost. Most people spend more time interacting through digital sources than they do through real life interactions – something that is beginning to take a toll on society.

Much of social media claims to be helping us with our lives – keeping us connected with the world around us and helping us stay "in the know" of what is going on in the lives of our friends and family. Unfortunately, this convenience has caused us to sign up for more social media accounts, follow more people, and subscribe to more updates than we know what to do with.

By going through your digital devices (and thus your portal into the digital world) you will have the opportunity to cut out a lot of the distractions that threaten to take over your mind and leave you with mental clutter. Going through your media devices will likely take as much effort as you spent going through your house, but trust me – you will be so happy you did when you are finally done.

To start, go through your phone and any other devices you may own. On a device by device level, clean up the things that you don't use.

This includes all the apps you don't use, all the things you signed up for "push notifications," and the songs you don't listen to. Once you have gone through all these things, flip through your contacts.

Are any of your contacts people you don't know or people you haven't spoken with since you can't remember when? Odds are it's time to get that contact go and focus on connecting with those you clearly do wish to keep in contact with. It's easy to delete a number and move on – just don't give it another thought.

If you have any music or apps that you wish to keep, but want to remove from your phone or other device, upload them into your storage cloud. This can be considered your digital storage closet – a place where you keep the things you truly do care about, but where those same things aren't in your face or taking up the space you wish to use.

After you have gone through your devices, it's time to take to the web and clean up the clutter that has accumulated there – trust me, you're going to be surprised at how many things you have allowed to slip into your life and take up your mental energy.

Start with your email inbox. How many emails do you receive that you never open? These can come from different department stores, online stores, or news updates that you signed up for when you were trying to learn a new hobby, but you never unsubscribed from when you lost interest in said hobby.

Unsubscribe from all the emails and updates you never read, and if you receive updates from solicitors, mark them as spam. You never have any real reason to enter your spam folder, so again, don't feel guilty about what goes in there. Mark it and forget it then move on with your day.

Following your email, it's time to tackle the social aspect of your digital world – social media.

Social media comes in many different forms. We often think of Twitter, Facebook, Instagram, and others like these when we think of social media, but any forum you read, any chat room you are a part of, or any vlog or blog you engage in are all forms of social media.

Go through the list of accounts you have, and close the accounts for the sites you don't visit. Just because it exists doesn't mean you have to be a part of it, and you'll find hanging out on the one or two sites you do enjoy is going to be a lot more fulfilling than bouncing around sites you don't enjoy just to see what is happening there.

There is nothing wrong with not being on a social media site. Though many people have the tendency to sign up and be a part of any and every new social media site that hits the web, few people actually spend time on any besides the ones they enjoy most. It's easy to get entrenched in a life full of gossip and trying to keep up with everything for the sake of things.

Cut back on your social media outlets drastically, then go through the accounts you wish to keep and declutter them so you are only seeing the things you really want to see.

Don't follow for the sake of following. If you aren't interested in something, don't follow it. Many people follow as many as possible, but end up scrolling through a feed that is so complex they rarely find much of what they really want to see. Unfollow those you don't care to watch, or hide them from your feed.

Leave the things you truly are interested in, and every time you get on your social media, your feed will be filled with only the things you truly care about. This is going to drastically change the way you feel about social media when you log on, and cut back on the stress you feel from seeing things you don't wish to see.

With the rise of social media came the rise of pressure – the rise to be popular among followers and friends, and the rise to perform as you think they want you to be. At the same time, people became so afraid they were going to miss out on something, they refuse to cut back or cut out social media they never use or aren't interested in.

Give yourself permission to not care or be consumed with the things that are going on in the screen of your device, and learn how to be comfortable with the life you are living – even if it means you miss out on some gossip that is taking place.

We as people aren't designed to be bombarded with that much information from that many people on a daily basis. By doing this to ourselves, we are only breeding more mental clutter where there really doesn't need to be any.

Chapter 7 – Clarity of Mind: Learning Mindfulness

The human brain is designed to constantly be filled with something. We are truly only able to focus on a single thing at a time, but while this is true, we are also designed to constantly be focusing on the things around us. Those who are good at multitasking have learned how to focus on many different things a little at a time, giving them the ability to get a lot done at the same time.

My point is that when you clear your mind of some things, you must be prepared to fill it with something else, or it won't be long and you will be drowning in mental clutter once again. Now, you may be thinking about how I said empty space has value, even when it is in your mind – and I am standing by that.

In this chapter, you are going to learn how to control your mind and fill it with the things you are currently doing. You are going to learn how to appreciate what the moment has to offer, and how to experience each moment fully. This is not only going to relax your body and remove stress, but it is also going to take up the bare space in your brain, making it impossible for mental clutter to move back in.

Mindfulness is the practice of being in the moment. It requires you to pay attention and appreciate your life as you are living it right now, and eliminates the worry about what is going on elsewhere – now or in the future.

One of the best ways to engage in mindfulness is through the practice of meditation. Meditation is the practice of clearing your mind and allowing yourself to simply *be*. Although many people have heard of meditation in their lives, few understand what it is or how to properly do it.

While you may have seen the stereotypical meditation in cartoons don't worry, that is not what you do to meditate. In fact, meditation can be done by merely lying on your back on the floor or sitting in a comfortable position and clearing your mind.

You can find countless guided meditations online, especially through sites such as YouTube. What's more is that you can decide how long you want your meditation session to be, and you can decide how much involvement you want from the instructor.

There are meditations available in which you choose the time and merely close your eyes as you listen to the calming music. These kinds of meditations allow you to guide yourself through the process, clearing your own mind, focusing on your own breathing, and letting your thoughts come without judgement of what those thoughts are. Some people respond very well to this form of meditation, and start their day in the right mindset.

Others, on the other hand, find it more difficult to focus on their meditation when they aren't being guided by an instructor. For these kinds of people, guided meditations are a better option. Again, you can choose the length of meditation you wish to participate in (which will allow you to better focus on the meditation rather than the clock) and whether you want to be guided visually or spiritually.

Regardless of the meditation you choose, you will want to relax yourself as much as possible. By relaxing and clearing your mind, you can focus on your breathing, and flooding your body with much-needed oxygen.

Focus on breathing out all the tension and negativity that builds up in your body, and draw in fresh, clean air.

If you are using a guided meditation, you will be instructed on how long to take a breath in, followed by how long to breathe it out again. Often, the instructor will count while you take your breath in, then count again as you breathe it out. The instructor will also tell you what part of your body to focus on, and how to guide your thoughts as you breathe.

It is remarkable how many incredible benefits come from the practice of meditation. Studies conducted all over the world have revealed that meditation causes real physical changes to take place in the brain – changes that make you better able to tolerate pain and stress, and put you in more control over your emotions.

Focus increases, as does the drive to get things done throughout the day. Those who meditate also report sleeping better at night and feeling refreshed when they wake up the next day.

But, perhaps the best benefit you will reap from your meditation comes in the fact that you will not feel nearly as stressed, and your mental clutter won't be coming back. You'll be able to face your day with a clarity of mind like never before.

Meditation is best done on a daily basis, and is even better when you can incorporate it into your day at least twice.

Studies have also shown that those who meditate for even 10 minute sessions twice a day experience incredible health benefits. Try it out for yourself before you get out of bed in the morning and before you go to bed at night – you just may be surprised at the host of health benefits that will flood your life.

Although meditation is huge in the mindfulness lifestyle, it's not the only part of the lifestyle. Being mindful means you also enjoy the little things in your life, allowing yourself to be in the moment fully.

As you eat your breakfast or your lunch, focus on how the food feels in your mouth. Focus on how it tastes. Think about how it makes you feel.

When you get dressed, really think about how the fabric feels against your skin, and how the brush feels as it runs through your hair. Think about how the sun and the breeze feel on your skin, and simply enjoy the moment for all it has to offer.

Mindfulness keeps you in the moment – ignoring all the excess things that turn into clutter in your brain. Today, starting right now, begin focusing on where you are and what you are doing – and only where you are and what you are doing.

Chapter 8 – The Art of Saying "No"

One of the biggest problems many people face in life – and one of the biggest sources of mental clutter – is the inability to say the word no. For any number of reasons, people are too scared to tell other people that they can't do what is being asked of them, and they end up overburdened and obligated to do things they don't wish to be doing.

One of the fastest and easiest ways you can clear yourself of mental clutter is to learn the art of saying no to the people around you, and sticking with what you have said.

To learn how to say no, it's best to first understand why you are always saying yes.

- **Do you feel guilty saying no?**
- **Are you scared they are going to get mad at you?**
- **Do you think they aren't going to like you anymore if you don't agree to do what they want you to do?**
- **Are you scared you are going to hurt someone else's feelings?**

- **Are you trying to be the popular one who is always there to do something whenever they are asked?**

If you were to be perfectly honest with yourself, it's likely the main reason you refuse to say no is out of fear. You don't want to lose social standing with someone. You don't want someone to get mad at you. You're scared you will be placed in some kind of uncomfortable situation, and worry that you won't be able to enjoy the level of social statues you are in right now.

But, as a result, you are constantly doing things you don't want to be doing, stressing yourself out over how you are going to make ends meet in your own life while fulfilling all these other obligations you have allowed yourself to become a part of, and you aren't happy with yourself for always saying yes.

At the same time, have you ever noticed that others don't have a problem saying no to you? Perhaps they do it in such a way that you don't even realize that they have, but you continue to say yes to everything everyone else wants.

If you are going to truly enjoy your newly found mental freedom, you are going to have to learn how to say the simply word, *no*.

Here are three different ways you can turn someone down without being rude – it's going to take practice before you master the art of doing it naturally, but trust me, practice makes perfect.

1. **"I'm sorry, that won't work for me."**

    This is the firm way of saying no. Whatever the request was, you don't want to be part of it, and you tell them up front that you can't. If you are pressed for a reason why, simply tell the person that it isn't going to fit into your schedule.

    Don't make excuses, don't try to fix it with some other offer – simply tell the individual that the idea isn't going to work for you, and move on with your day.

2. **"Let me think about it, and I will get back to you with an answer."**

    If you don't feel like you are ready to simply tell someone no, ask them for some time. Give yourself time to work up the courage to turn them down (just make sure you stick with your guns and actually turn them down.)

    If they press you for an answer right then and right there, tell them you're going to have to say no, because you don't agree to doing things when you are under pressure. When you let go of the need to explain things, or the need to have the approval of everyone, you free yourself to say how you truly feel about a situation.

Yes, this is something that is very scary for some people, but again, practice makes perfect.

3. **"I'm sorry, I won't be able to commit to that, but I would be able to ________"**

There may be times in your life when you do want to be a part of something, but you aren't able to commit to the level of work a person is asking you to do.

For example, if you were asked to help plan a party, but you don't feel you have the time to properly plan, you could say something like, "I'm sorry, I won't be able to commit to planning the party, but I would love to be in charge of bringing the cake."

You tell the individual no, and you free yourself from doing the things you don't wish to do. At the same time, you do offer to still be a part of the occasion, and you offer to do something that will help, though it's not at the same level of commitment they were asking of you.

Saying "no" is a delicate dance for a lot of people, because they really don't want to be rude. However, when you turn someone down, it is important that you do it properly, and that you stick with your guns.

Don't ever be rude. There is always a nice way to do something, even if you are in a tense situation. Always be polite and respectful, but be kind and firm in what you say. At the same time, don't try to be the hero. You said no, now it is up to them to figure out an alternative.

Also, never offer explanations beyond "that doesn't work for my schedule" because by offering an explanation, you are then giving that person the opportunity to decide whether your reason for saying no is a good enough reason or not. Just turn them down as graciously as possible, don't offer explanations, and don't feel guilty about declining.

By learning this art, you are going to give yourself so much freedom in your schedule – the stress really will melt away.

Chapter 9 – How to Teach an Old Mind New Tricks

If there is one thing I want you to learn through these chapters, it is that mental clutter is a habit, and you can change your habits. Many people feel that they are stuck in life – stuck in their circumstances, stuck with their problems, stuck with the people they know – but they are wrong.

There are very few things in your life that can't be changed, and that is crucial to remember as you sift through this mental clutter. Always know that you are able to change what is happening to you, or the things you are doing. Always.

Don't allow your brain to tell you that you are stuck, or that there are things you can't do for yourself. Regardless of your situation, you will always be able to make changes you wish to make.

I'm not saying that it's going to be easy, and I'm not saying that you aren't going to have some days that are worse than others. What I really want you to hear, however, is that you will push through, and you will begin to see the results you are hoping for if you don't give up.

Our minds are able to grow and change in incredible ways, and just as the mental clutter slipped in unnoticed, you won't notice the subtle changes until they become habits that make you feel on top of the world. Take each day as a new opportunity to do better, then truly do better.

Each moment of each day you have the decision to be the person you wish to be, or to stay stuck as the person you are unhappy with. Don't let your brain – or anyone else – tell you that you aren't able to change. Clear your mental clutter, and you will realize how to live life to the fullest.

It's a matter of choice – one minute at a time.

Conclusion

There you have it, everything you need to know to declutter your mind and get yourself on the right track to mental healing. I hope this book was able to inspire you to get rid of all those extra things that weigh down on your mentality, and that you break free of the stress and complications that accompany worry.

This is a process, and it is going to take both time and effort on your part to conquer this habit and set your mind on the right track. But, just as slipping into mental clutter is a habit, breaking out of it is something you can learn to do, too.

You will have good days, and you will have bad days – the important thing is that you stick with it no matter what kind of day you're having. Habits take time to break, and new habits take time to form. As long as you are consistent and positive, you'll see the change take place naturally.

I hope you were able to glean practical, real applications from this book and insert them into your own life. Everyone's situation is unique, but these methods are certain to work for everyone as long as they are used consistently and diligently.

Mental clutter takes root deeply, and it is highly resistant to leaving. However, your mind allowed the clutter to build up in the first place, and it is strong enough to rid itself of the clutter if you focus on eliminating the problem. Cut off the issues at their roots – get rid of the clutter in your home, in your relationships, and in your social media.

Give yourself the permission to say no to people, and allow yourself to live in a guilt free manner. Embrace the ancient art of meditation, and open your mind to a whole new world of peace and tranquility. We live in a modern world that should be easier than ever, yet we choose to put ourselves under such stress that we crumble and fall under our own pressure.

Let this book change your life, and get rid of the clutter that threatens to ruin your happiness and your health. Remember that no matter how hard things get, you do have the power to change, and you are strong enough to maintain that change regardless of the outside circumstances you are dealing with.

Stay positive, and stick to your new mindset like it's the only way you've ever thought. Stress-free happiness is just around the corner – you just need to stick with it until it's a reality.

Good luck, and may you live a life of peace and happiness.